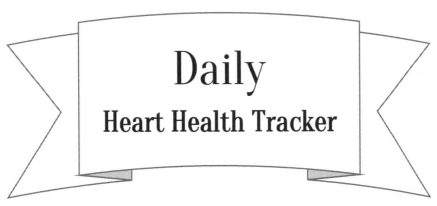

Daily
Heart Health Tracker

IMPORTANT MEDICAL CONTACTS

Name or Organization	Phone #

DISCLAIMER

This Daily Heart Health Tracker was developed as a convenient tool to record daily measurements related to heart health.

This information is not intended to diagnose health problems or to take the place of medical advice or care you receive from your physician or other health care professional. If you have persistent health problems, or if you have additional questions, please consult with your doctor.

Make Tracking A Daily Habit

People who have heart failure need to track their weight carefully. It is very important to check and record it every day.

When a situation gets worse in small steps, it's easy to not notice the changes as they happen Your sense of what is normal adjusts with the slow changes until you aren't really aware of what "normal" should be.

Checking your weight daily lets you know how much extra fluid your body is holding on to. Sudden weight gain may mean that your heart failure is getting worse. Tracking your daily weight changes is an important tool for you and your doctor to manage your heart disease.

How To Use This Log

- ✓ Keep this heart health log and a pen or pencil by your scale.
- ✓ Take this Daily Heart Health Log with you to every doctor's appointment you have.

When To Weigh Yourself

- ✓ Weigh yourself every morning after you empty your bladder, but before you eat breakfast.
- ✓ Try to weigh yourself around the same time every day

How To Weigh Yourself

- ✓ Weigh yourself without clothing on each day. If you must wear clothing, be sure to wear the same amount of clothing every time.
- ✓ Do not wear shoes when you weigh yourself.

About The Scale

- ✓ Use the same scale each time you weigh yourself. Make sure it is on a hard surface, not on carpet.
- ✓ Set the scale to zero before weighing yourself.

When To Call 911

If you experience any of these **emergency symptoms*** of heart failure, immediately call 9-1-1 or go to the nearest hospital emergency room:

- Severe shortness of breath with or without chest discomfort
- Coughing up pink, frothy sputum
- Fainting, passing out, or extreme dizziness
- Feeling confused or that you can't think clearly
- Chest discomfort, fullness, pain, or pressure not relieved by rest or by taking nitroglycerin (if it is prescribed for you) that lasts more than a few minutes or goes away and comes back.
- Pain or discomfort in one or both arms, the back, neck, jaw or stomach.
- Other signs such as breaking out in a cold sweat, nausea or lightheadedness.
- **Special Note for Women:** As with men, women's most common heart attack symptom is chest pain or discomfort. But women are somewhat more likely than men to experience some of the other common symptoms, particularly:
    - shortness of breath,
    - a feeling of heartburn/indigestion,
    - nausea/vomiting,
    - neck, back or jaw pain.

    Often, women experience heart attacks as pain in the center of their back that is mistaken for back strain or other issues. Signs of a heart attack for women may be less obvious than for men. Women are quick to disregard these signs and explain them away as something else. Don't make that mistake. If it feels "wrong", then it probably is.

---

* PLEASE NOTE: An *Emergency Medical Condition* is defined by the Emergency Medical Treatment and Labor Act (EMTALA) as "a condition manifesting itself by acute symptoms of sufficient severity (including severe pain) such that you could reasonably expect the absence of immediate medical attention to result in serious jeopardy to your health or serious impairment or dysfunction of your bodily functions or organs."

When To Call Your Doctor

Call your physician or other health care professional right away if the following symptoms get worse or if they are new for you:

- **Sudden weight gain.** As a rule of thumb, call your doctor if you gain two or more pounds in one day, more than one pound each day for three days in a row, or five or more pounds gained in one week.
- **Change in blood pressure.**
- **Changes in your heart rate.** New or increasing irregularities in your heart rate.
- **Shortness of breath.** Do you have to stop to catch your breath during your daily activities such as getting dressed or climbing the stairs? This could be a sign of fluid buildup.
- **Swelling or water retention.** As you put your socks on in the morning check your ankles. Press your legs with your thumb – if it leaves an imprint there may be fluid. Contact your doctor if you notice increased swelling of your feet, legs, or abdominal area.
- **Difficulty breathing when you lie down flat.** You might find you need more pillows or a recliner to sleep at night. Tell your doctor if you are having to prop yourself up at night to breathe.
- **Breathing issues when sleeping.** If you wake up in the night feeling out of breath, or because you are panting or breathing rapidly, contact your doctor.
- **Dizziness or falling.** New or worsening dizziness and/or lightheadedness, fainting, or loss of consciousness. Falls can be caused by a loss of consciousness that isn't remembered later.
- **A cough that does not go away.**
- **Any problems with your medications.**
- **Feeling uneasy.** If you have a sense that something just isn't "right", trust your instincts and call your doctor. Also, pay attention to new or worsening sadness or depression.

WEEK OF:

	Date & Time	Today's Weight	B.P.	Heart Rate	Blood Sugar Measurements (mg/dL)
MON		lbs	—	beats per minute	
TUE		lbs	—	beats per minute	
WED	2/17	lbs	—	62 beats per minute	
THU		lbs	—	beats per minute	
FRI		lbs	—	beats per minute	
SAT		lbs	—	beats per minute	
SUN		lbs	—	beats per minute	

	Meds Taken (Y/N)	Daily Activity & Duration	Note if you are experiencing any symptoms listed on page 5: "When To Call Your Doctor"
MON			
TUE			
WED			
THU			
FRI			
SAT			
SUN			

WEEK OF:

	Date & Time	Today's Weight	B.P.	Heart Rate	Blood Sugar Measurements (mg/dL)
MON		lbs	—	beats per minute	
TUE		lbs	—	beats per minute	
WED		lbs	—	beats per minute	
THU		lbs	—	beats per minute	
FRI		lbs	—	beats per minute	
SAT		lbs	—	beats per minute	
SUN		lbs	—	beats per minute	

	Meds Taken (Y/N)	Daily Activity & Duration	Note if you are experiencing any symptoms listed on page 5: "When To Call Your Doctor"
MON			
TUE			
WED			
THU			
FRI			
SAT			
SUN			

WEEK OF:

	Date & Time	Today's Weight	B.P.	Heart Rate	Blood Sugar Measurements (mg/dL)
MON		lbs	—	beats per minute	
TUE		lbs	—	beats per minute	
WED		lbs	—	beats per minute	
THU		lbs	—	beats per minute	
FRI		lbs	—	beats per minute	
SAT		lbs	—	beats per minute	
SUN		lbs	—	beats per minute	

	Meds Taken (Y/N)	Daily Activity & Duration	Note if you are experiencing any symptoms listed on page 5: "When To Call Your Doctor"
MON			
TUE			
WED			
THU			
FRI			
SAT			
SUN			

WEEK OF:

	Date & Time	Today's Weight	B.P.	Heart Rate	Blood Sugar Measurements (mg/dL)
MON		lbs	—	beats per minute	
TUE		lbs	—	beats per minute	
WED		lbs	—	beats per minute	
THU		lbs	—	beats per minute	
FRI		lbs	—	beats per minute	
SAT		lbs	—	beats per minute	
SUN		lbs	—	beats per minute	

	Meds Taken (Y/N)	Daily Activity & Duration	Note if you are experiencing any symptoms listed on page 5: "When To Call Your Doctor"
MON			
TUE			
WED			
THU			
FRI			
SAT			
SUN			

WEEK OF:

	Date & Time	Today's Weight	B.P.	Heart Rate	Blood Sugar Measurements (mg/dL)
MON		lbs	—	beats per minute	
TUE		lbs	—	beats per minute	
WED		lbs	—	beats per minute	
THU		lbs	—	beats per minute	
FRI		lbs	—	beats per minute	
SAT		lbs	—	beats per minute	
SUN		lbs	—	beats per minute	

	Meds Taken (Y/N)	Daily Activity & Duration	Note if you are experiencing any symptoms listed on page 5: "When To Call Your Doctor"
MON			
TUE			
WED			
THU			
FRI			
SAT			
SUN			

WEEK OF:

	Date & Time	Today's Weight	B.P.	Heart Rate	Blood Sugar Measurements (mg/dL)
MON		lbs	—	beats per minute	
TUE		lbs	—	beats per minute	
WED		lbs	—	beats per minute	
THU		lbs	—	beats per minute	
FRI		lbs	—	beats per minute	
SAT		lbs	—	beats per minute	
SUN		lbs	—	beats per minute	

	Meds Taken (Y/N)	Daily Activity & Duration	Note if you are experiencing any symptoms listed on page 5: "When To Call Your Doctor"
MON			
TUE			
WED			
THU			
FRI			
SAT			
SUN			

WEEK OF:

	Date & Time	Today's Weight	B.P.	Heart Rate	Blood Sugar Measurements (mg/dL)
MON		lbs	—	beats per minute	
TUE		lbs	—	beats per minute	
WED		lbs	—	beats per minute	
THU		lbs	—	beats per minute	
FRI		lbs	—	beats per minute	
SAT		lbs	—	beats per minute	
SUN		lbs	—	beats per minute	

	Meds Taken (Y/N)	Daily Activity & Duration	Note if you are experiencing any symptoms listed on page 5: "When To Call Your Doctor"
MON			
TUE			
WED			
THU			
FRI			
SAT			
SUN			

WEEK OF:

	Date & Time	Today's Weight	B.P.	Heart Rate	Blood Sugar Measurements (mg/dL)
MON		lbs	—	beats per minute	
TUE		lbs	—	beats per minute	
WED		lbs	—	beats per minute	
THU		lbs	—	beats per minute	
FRI		lbs	—	beats per minute	
SAT		lbs	—	beats per minute	
SUN		lbs	—	beats per minute	

	Meds Taken (Y/N)	Daily Activity & Duration	Note if you are experiencing any symptoms listed on page 5: "When To Call Your Doctor"
MON			
TUE			
WED			
THU			
FRI			
SAT			
SUN			

WEEK OF:

	Date & Time	Today's Weight	B.P.	Heart Rate	Blood Sugar Measurements (mg/dL)
MON		lbs	—	beats per minute	
TUE		lbs	—	beats per minute	
WED		lbs	—	beats per minute	
THU		lbs	—	beats per minute	
FRI		lbs	—	beats per minute	
SAT		lbs	—	beats per minute	
SUN		lbs	—	beats per minute	

	Meds Taken (Y/N)	Daily Activity & Duration	Note if you are experiencing any symptoms listed on page 5: "When To Call Your Doctor"
MON			
TUE			
WED			
THU			
FRI			
SAT			
SUN			

WEEK OF:

	Date & Time	Today's Weight	B.P.	Heart Rate	Blood Sugar Measurements (mg/dL)
MON		lbs	—	beats per minute	
TUE		lbs	—	beats per minute	
WED		lbs	—	beats per minute	
THU		lbs	—	beats per minute	
FRI		lbs	—	beats per minute	
SAT		lbs	—	beats per minute	
SUN		lbs	—	beats per minute	

	Meds Taken (Y/N)	Daily Activity & Duration	Note if you are experiencing any symptoms listed on page 5: "When To Call Your Doctor"
MON			
TUE			
WED			
THU			
FRI			
SAT			
SUN			

WEEK OF:

	Date & Time	Today's Weight	B.P.	Heart Rate	Blood Sugar Measurements (mg/dL)
MON		lbs	—	beats per minute	
TUE		lbs	—	beats per minute	
WED		lbs	—	beats per minute	
THU		lbs	—	beats per minute	
FRI		lbs	—	beats per minute	
SAT		lbs	—	beats per minute	
SUN		lbs	—	beats per minute	

	Meds Taken (Y/N)	Daily Activity & Duration	Note if you are experiencing any symptoms listed on page 5: "When To Call Your Doctor"
MON			
TUE			
WED			
THU			
FRI			
SAT			
SUN			

WEEK OF:

	Date & Time	Today's Weight	B.P.	Heart Rate	Blood Sugar Measurements (mg/dL)
MON		lbs	—	beats per minute	
TUE		lbs	—	beats per minute	
WED		lbs	—	beats per minute	
THU		lbs	—	beats per minute	
FRI		lbs	—	beats per minute	
SAT		lbs	—	beats per minute	
SUN		lbs	—	beats per minute	

	Meds Taken (Y/N)	Daily Activity & Duration	Note if you are experiencing any symptoms listed on page 5: "When To Call Your Doctor"
MON			
TUE			
WED			
THU			
FRI			
SAT			
SUN			

WEEK OF:

	Date & Time	Today's Weight	B.P.	Heart Rate	Blood Sugar Measurements (mg/dL)
MON		lbs	—	beats per minute	
TUE		lbs	—	beats per minute	
WED		lbs	—	beats per minute	
THU		lbs	—	beats per minute	
FRI		lbs	—	beats per minute	
SAT		lbs	—	beats per minute	
SUN		lbs	—	beats per minute	

	Meds Taken (Y/N)	Daily Activity & Duration	Note if you are experiencing any symptoms listed on page 5: "When To Call Your Doctor"
MON			
TUE			
WED			
THU			
FRI			
SAT			
SUN			

WEEK OF:

	Date & Time	Today's Weight	B.P.	Heart Rate	Blood Sugar Measurements (mg/dL)
MON		lbs	—	beats per minute	
TUE		lbs	—	beats per minute	
WED		lbs	—	beats per minute	
THU		lbs	—	beats per minute	
FRI		lbs	—	beats per minute	
SAT		lbs	—	beats per minute	
SUN		lbs	—	beats per minute	

	Meds Taken (Y/N)	Daily Activity & Duration	Note if you are experiencing any symptoms listed on page 5: "When To Call Your Doctor"
MON			
TUE			
WED			
THU			
FRI			
SAT			
SUN			

WEEK OF:

	Date & Time	Today's Weight	B.P.	Heart Rate	Blood Sugar Measurements (mg/dL)
MON		lbs	—	beats per minute	
TUE		lbs	—	beats per minute	
WED		lbs	—	beats per minute	
THU		lbs	—	beats per minute	
FRI		lbs	—	beats per minute	
SAT		lbs	—	beats per minute	
SUN		lbs	—	beats per minute	

	Meds Taken (Y/N)	Daily Activity & Duration	Note if you are experiencing any symptoms listed on page 5: "When To Call Your Doctor"
MON			
TUE			
WED			
THU			
FRI			
SAT			
SUN			

WEEK OF:

	Date & Time	Today's Weight	B.P.	Heart Rate	Blood Sugar Measurements (mg/dL)
MON		lbs	—	beats per minute	
TUE		lbs	—	beats per minute	
WED		lbs	—	beats per minute	
THU		lbs	—	beats per minute	
FRI		lbs	—	beats per minute	
SAT		lbs	—	beats per minute	
SUN		lbs	—	beats per minute	

	Meds Taken (Y/N)	Daily Activity & Duration	Note if you are experiencing any symptoms listed on page 5: "When To Call Your Doctor"
MON			
TUE			
WED			
THU			
FRI			
SAT			
SUN			

WEEK OF:

	Date & Time	Today's Weight	B.P.	Heart Rate	Blood Sugar Measurements (mg/dL)
MON		lbs	—	beats per minute	
TUE		lbs	—	beats per minute	
WED		lbs	—	beats per minute	
THU		lbs	—	beats per minute	
FRI		lbs	—	beats per minute	
SAT		lbs	—	beats per minute	
SUN		lbs	—	beats per minute	

	Meds Taken (Y/N)	Daily Activity & Duration	Note if you are experiencing any symptoms listed on page 5: "When To Call Your Doctor"
MON			
TUE			
WED			
THU			
FRI			
SAT			
SUN			

WEEK OF:

	Date & Time	Today's Weight	B.P.	Heart Rate	Blood Sugar Measurements (mg/dL)
MON		lbs	—	beats per minute	
TUE		lbs	—	beats per minute	
WED		lbs	—	beats per minute	
THU		lbs	—	beats per minute	
FRI		lbs	—	beats per minute	
SAT		lbs	—	beats per minute	
SUN		lbs	—	beats per minute	

	Meds Taken (Y/N)	Daily Activity & Duration	Note if you are experiencing any symptoms listed on page 5: "When To Call Your Doctor"
MON			
TUE			
WED			
THU			
FRI			
SAT			
SUN			

WEEK OF:

	Date & Time	Today's Weight	B.P.	Heart Rate	Blood Sugar Measurements (mg/dL)
MON		lbs	—	beats per minute	
TUE		lbs	—	beats per minute	
WED		lbs	—	beats per minute	
THU		lbs	—	beats per minute	
FRI		lbs	—	beats per minute	
SAT		lbs	—	beats per minute	
SUN		lbs	—	beats per minute	

	Meds Taken (Y/N)	Daily Activity & Duration	Note if you are experiencing any symptoms listed on page 5: "When To Call Your Doctor"
MON			
TUE			
WED			
THU			
FRI			
SAT			
SUN			

WEEK OF:

	Date & Time	Today's Weight	B.P.	Heart Rate	Blood Sugar Measurements (mg/dL)
MON		lbs	—	beats per minute	
TUE		lbs	—	beats per minute	
WED		lbs	—	beats per minute	
THU		lbs	—	beats per minute	
FRI		lbs	—	beats per minute	
SAT		lbs	—	beats per minute	
SUN		lbs	—	beats per minute	

	Meds Taken (Y/N)	Daily Activity & Duration	Note if you are experiencing any symptoms listed on page 5: "When To Call Your Doctor"
MON			
TUE			
WED			
THU			
FRI			
SAT			
SUN			

WEEK OF:

	Date & Time	Today's Weight	B.P.	Heart Rate	Blood Sugar Measurements (mg/dL)
MON		lbs	—	beats per minute	
TUE		lbs	—	beats per minute	
WED		lbs	—	beats per minute	
THU		lbs	—	beats per minute	
FRI		lbs	—	beats per minute	
SAT		lbs	—	beats per minute	
SUN		lbs	—	beats per minute	

	Meds Taken (Y/N)	Daily Activity & Duration	Note if you are experiencing any symptoms listed on page 5: "When To Call Your Doctor"
MON			
TUE			
WED			
THU			
FRI			
SAT			
SUN			

WEEK OF:

	Date & Time	Today's Weight	B.P.	Heart Rate	Blood Sugar Measurements (mg/dL)
MON		lbs	—	beats per minute	
TUE		lbs	—	beats per minute	
WED		lbs	—	beats per minute	
THU		lbs	—	beats per minute	
FRI		lbs	—	beats per minute	
SAT		lbs	—	beats per minute	
SUN		lbs	—	beats per minute	

	Meds Taken (Y/N)	Daily Activity & Duration	Note if you are experiencing any symptoms listed on page 5: "When To Call Your Doctor"
MON			
TUE			
WED			
THU			
FRI			
SAT			
SUN			

WEEK OF:

	Date & Time	Today's Weight	B.P.	Heart Rate	Blood Sugar Measurements (mg/dL)
MON		lbs	—	beats per minute	
TUE		lbs	—	beats per minute	
WED		lbs	—	beats per minute	
THU		lbs	—	beats per minute	
FRI		lbs	—	beats per minute	
SAT		lbs	—	beats per minute	
SUN		lbs	—	beats per minute	

	Meds Taken (Y/N)	Daily Activity & Duration	Note if you are experiencing any symptoms listed on page 5: "When To Call Your Doctor"
MON			
TUE			
WED			
THU			
FRI			
SAT			
SUN			

WEEK OF:

	Date & Time	Today's Weight	B.P.	Heart Rate	Blood Sugar Measurements (mg/dL)
MON		lbs	—	beats per minute	
TUE		lbs	—	beats per minute	
WED		lbs	—	beats per minute	
THU		lbs	—	beats per minute	
FRI		lbs	—	beats per minute	
SAT		lbs	—	beats per minute	
SUN		lbs	—	beats per minute	

	Meds Taken (Y/N)	Daily Activity & Duration	Note if you are experiencing any symptoms listed on page 5: "When To Call Your Doctor"
MON			
TUE			
WED			
THU			
FRI			
SAT			
SUN			

WEEK OF:

	Date & Time	Today's Weight	B.P.	Heart Rate	Blood Sugar Measurements (mg/dL)
MON		lbs	—	beats per minute	
TUE		lbs	—	beats per minute	
WED		lbs	—	beats per minute	
THU		lbs	—	beats per minute	
FRI		lbs	—	beats per minute	
SAT		lbs	—	beats per minute	
SUN		lbs	—	beats per minute	

	Meds Taken (Y/N)	Daily Activity & Duration	Note if you are experiencing any symptoms listed on page 5: "When To Call Your Doctor"
MON			
TUE			
WED			
THU			
FRI			
SAT			
SUN			

WEEK OF:

	Date & Time	Today's Weight	B.P.	Heart Rate	Blood Sugar Measurements (mg/dL)
MON		lbs	—	beats per minute	
TUE		lbs	—	beats per minute	
WED		lbs	—	beats per minute	
THU		lbs	—	beats per minute	
FRI		lbs	—	beats per minute	
SAT		lbs	—	beats per minute	
SUN		lbs	—	beats per minute	

	Meds Taken (Y/N)	Daily Activity & Duration	Note if you are experiencing any symptoms listed on page 5: "When To Call Your Doctor"
MON			
TUE			
WED			
THU			
FRI			
SAT			
SUN			

WEEK OF:

	Date & Time	Today's Weight	B.P.	Heart Rate	Blood Sugar Measurements (mg/dL)
MON		lbs	—	beats per minute	
TUE		lbs	—	beats per minute	
WED		lbs	—	beats per minute	
THU		lbs	—	beats per minute	
FRI		lbs	—	beats per minute	
SAT		lbs	—	beats per minute	
SUN		lbs	—	beats per minute	

	Meds Taken (Y/N)	Daily Activity & Duration	Note if you are experiencing any symptoms listed on page 5: "When To Call Your Doctor"
MON			
TUE			
WED			
THU			
FRI			
SAT			
SUN			

WEEK OF:

	Date & Time	Today's Weight	B.P.	Heart Rate	Blood Sugar Measurements (mg/dL)
MON		lbs	—	beats per minute	
TUE		lbs	—	beats per minute	
WED		lbs	—	beats per minute	
THU		lbs	—	beats per minute	
FRI		lbs	—	beats per minute	
SAT		lbs	—	beats per minute	
SUN		lbs	—	beats per minute	

	Meds Taken (Y/N)	Daily Activity & Duration	Note if you are experiencing any symptoms listed on page 5: "When To Call Your Doctor"
MON			
TUE			
WED			
THU			
FRI			
SAT			
SUN			

WEEK OF:

	Date & Time	Today's Weight	B.P.	Heart Rate	Blood Sugar Measurements (mg/dL)
MON		lbs	—	beats per minute	
TUE		lbs	—	beats per minute	
WED		lbs	—	beats per minute	
THU		lbs	—	beats per minute	
FRI		lbs	—	beats per minute	
SAT		lbs	—	beats per minute	
SUN		lbs	—	beats per minute	

	Meds Taken (Y/N)	Daily Activity & Duration	Note if you are experiencing any symptoms listed on page 5: "When To Call Your Doctor"
MON			
TUE			
WED			
THU			
FRI			
SAT			
SUN			

WEEK OF:

	Date & Time	Today's Weight	B.P.	Heart Rate	Blood Sugar Measurements (mg/dL)
MON		lbs	—	beats per minute	
TUE		lbs	—	beats per minute	
WED		lbs	—	beats per minute	
THU		lbs	—	beats per minute	
FRI		lbs	—	beats per minute	
SAT		lbs	—	beats per minute	
SUN		lbs	—	beats per minute	

	Meds Taken (Y/N)	Daily Activity & Duration	Note if you are experiencing any symptoms listed on page 5: "When To Call Your Doctor"
MON			
TUE			
WED			
THU			
FRI			
SAT			
SUN			

WEEK OF:

	Date & Time	Today's Weight	B.P.	Heart Rate	Blood Sugar Measurements (mg/dL)
MON		lbs	—	beats per minute	
TUE		lbs	—	beats per minute	
WED		lbs	—	beats per minute	
THU		lbs	—	beats per minute	
FRI		lbs	—	beats per minute	
SAT		lbs	—	beats per minute	
SUN		lbs	—	beats per minute	

	Meds Taken (Y/N)	Daily Activity & Duration	Note if you are experiencing any symptoms listed on page 5: "When To Call Your Doctor"
MON			
TUE			
WED			
THU			
FRI			
SAT			
SUN			

WEEK OF:

	Date & Time	Today's Weight	B.P.	Heart Rate	Blood Sugar Measurements (mg/dL)
MON		lbs	—	beats per minute	
TUE		lbs	—	beats per minute	
WED		lbs	—	beats per minute	
THU		lbs	—	beats per minute	
FRI		lbs	—	beats per minute	
SAT		lbs	—	beats per minute	
SUN		lbs	—	beats per minute	

	Meds Taken (Y/N)	Daily Activity & Duration	Note if you are experiencing any symptoms listed on page 5: "When To Call Your Doctor"
MON			
TUE			
WED			
THU			
FRI			
SAT			
SUN			

WEEK OF:

	Date & Time	Today's Weight	B.P.	Heart Rate	Blood Sugar Measurements (mg/dL)
MON		lbs	—	beats per minute	
TUE		lbs	—	beats per minute	
WED		lbs	—	beats per minute	
THU		lbs	—	beats per minute	
FRI		lbs	—	beats per minute	
SAT		lbs	—	beats per minute	
SUN		lbs	—	beats per minute	

	Meds Taken (Y/N)	Daily Activity & Duration	Note if you are experiencing any symptoms listed on page 5: "When To Call Your Doctor"
MON			
TUE			
WED			
THU			
FRI			
SAT			
SUN			

WEEK OF:

	Date & Time	Today's Weight	B.P.	Heart Rate	Blood Sugar Measurements (mg/dL)
MON		lbs	—	beats per minute	
TUE		lbs	—	beats per minute	
WED		lbs	—	beats per minute	
THU		lbs	—	beats per minute	
FRI		lbs	—	beats per minute	
SAT		lbs	—	beats per minute	
SUN		lbs	—	beats per minute	

	Meds Taken (Y/N)	Daily Activity & Duration	Note if you are experiencing any symptoms listed on page 5: "When To Call Your Doctor"
MON			
TUE			
WED			
THU			
FRI			
SAT			
SUN			

WEEK OF:

	Date & Time	Today's Weight	B.P.	Heart Rate	Blood Sugar Measurements (mg/dL)
MON		lbs	—	beats per minute	
TUE		lbs	—	beats per minute	
WED		lbs	—	beats per minute	
THU		lbs	—	beats per minute	
FRI		lbs	—	beats per minute	
SAT		lbs	—	beats per minute	
SUN		lbs	—	beats per minute	

	Meds Taken (Y/N)	Daily Activity & Duration	Note if you are experiencing any symptoms listed on page 5: "When To Call Your Doctor"
MON			
TUE			
WED			
THU			
FRI			
SAT			
SUN			

WEEK OF:

	Date & Time	Today's Weight	B.P.	Heart Rate	Blood Sugar Measurements (mg/dL)
MON		lbs	—	beats per minute	
TUE		lbs	—	beats per minute	
WED		lbs	—	beats per minute	
THU		lbs	—	beats per minute	
FRI		lbs	—	beats per minute	
SAT		lbs	—	beats per minute	
SUN		lbs	—	beats per minute	

	Meds Taken (Y/N)	Daily Activity & Duration	Note if you are experiencing any symptoms listed on page 5: "When To Call Your Doctor"
MON			
TUE			
WED			
THU			
FRI			
SAT			
SUN			

WEEK OF:

	Date & Time	Today's Weight	B.P.	Heart Rate	Blood Sugar Measurements (mg/dL)
MON		lbs	—	beats per minute	
TUE		lbs	—	beats per minute	
WED		lbs	—	beats per minute	
THU		lbs	—	beats per minute	
FRI		lbs	—	beats per minute	
SAT		lbs	—	beats per minute	
SUN		lbs	—	beats per minute	

	Meds Taken (Y/N)	Daily Activity & Duration	Note if you are experiencing any symptoms listed on page 5: "When To Call Your Doctor"
MON			
TUE			
WED			
THU			
FRI			
SAT			
SUN			

WEEK OF:

	Date & Time	Today's Weight	B.P.	Heart Rate	Blood Sugar Measurements (mg/dL)
MON		lbs	—	beats per minute	
TUE		lbs	—	beats per minute	
WED		lbs	—	beats per minute	
THU		lbs	—	beats per minute	
FRI		lbs	—	beats per minute	
SAT		lbs	—	beats per minute	
SUN		lbs	—	beats per minute	

	Meds Taken (Y/N)	Daily Activity & Duration	Note if you are experiencing any symptoms listed on page 5: "When To Call Your Doctor"
MON			
TUE			
WED			
THU			
FRI			
SAT			
SUN			

WEEK OF:

	Date & Time	Today's Weight	B.P.	Heart Rate	Blood Sugar Measurements (mg/dL)
MON		lbs	—	beats per minute	
TUE		lbs	—	beats per minute	
WED		lbs	—	beats per minute	
THU		lbs	—	beats per minute	
FRI		lbs	—	beats per minute	
SAT		lbs	—	beats per minute	
SUN		lbs	—	beats per minute	

	Meds Taken (Y/N)	Daily Activity & Duration	Note if you are experiencing any symptoms listed on page 5: "When To Call Your Doctor"
MON			
TUE			
WED			
THU			
FRI			
SAT			
SUN			

WEEK OF:

	Date & Time	Today's Weight	B.P.	Heart Rate	Blood Sugar Measurements (mg/dL)
MON		lbs	—	beats per minute	
TUE		lbs	—	beats per minute	
WED		lbs	—	beats per minute	
THU		lbs	—	beats per minute	
FRI		lbs	—	beats per minute	
SAT		lbs	—	beats per minute	
SUN		lbs	—	beats per minute	

	Meds Taken (Y/N)	Daily Activity & Duration	Note if you are experiencing any symptoms listed on page 5: "When To Call Your Doctor"
MON			
TUE			
WED			
THU			
FRI			
SAT			
SUN			

WEEK OF:

	Date & Time	Today's Weight	B.P.	Heart Rate	Blood Sugar Measurements (mg/dL)
MON		lbs	—	beats per minute	
TUE		lbs	—	beats per minute	
WED		lbs	—	beats per minute	
THU		lbs	—	beats per minute	
FRI		lbs	—	beats per minute	
SAT		lbs	—	beats per minute	
SUN		lbs	—	beats per minute	

	Meds Taken (Y/N)	Daily Activity & Duration	Note if you are experiencing any symptoms listed on page 5: "When To Call Your Doctor"
MON			
TUE			
WED			
THU			
FRI			
SAT			
SUN			

WEEK OF:

	Date & Time	Today's Weight	B.P.	Heart Rate	Blood Sugar Measurements (mg/dL)
MON		lbs	—	beats per minute	
TUE		lbs	—	beats per minute	
WED		lbs	—	beats per minute	
THU		lbs	—	beats per minute	
FRI		lbs	—	beats per minute	
SAT		lbs	—	beats per minute	
SUN		lbs	—	beats per minute	

	Meds Taken (Y/N)	Daily Activity & Duration	Note if you are experiencing any symptoms listed on page 5: "When To Call Your Doctor"
MON			
TUE			
WED			
THU			
FRI			
SAT			
SUN			

WEEK OF:

	Date & Time	Today's Weight	B.P.	Heart Rate	Blood Sugar Measurements (mg/dL)
MON		lbs	—	beats per minute	
TUE		lbs	—	beats per minute	
WED		lbs	—	beats per minute	
THU		lbs	—	beats per minute	
FRI		lbs	—	beats per minute	
SAT		lbs	—	beats per minute	
SUN		lbs	—	beats per minute	

	Meds Taken (Y/N)	Daily Activity & Duration	Note if you are experiencing any symptoms listed on page 5: "When To Call Your Doctor"
MON			
TUE			
WED			
THU			
FRI			
SAT			
SUN			

WEEK OF:

	Date & Time	Today's Weight	B.P.	Heart Rate	Blood Sugar Measurements (mg/dL)
MON		lbs	—	beats per minute	
TUE		lbs	—	beats per minute	
WED		lbs	—	beats per minute	
THU		lbs	—	beats per minute	
FRI		lbs	—	beats per minute	
SAT		lbs	—	beats per minute	
SUN		lbs	—	beats per minute	

	Meds Taken (Y/N)	Daily Activity & Duration	Note if you are experiencing any symptoms listed on page 5: "When To Call Your Doctor"
MON			
TUE			
WED			
THU			
FRI			
SAT			
SUN			

WEEK OF:

	Date & Time	Today's Weight	B.P.	Heart Rate	Blood Sugar Measurements (mg/dL)
MON		lbs	—	beats per minute	
TUE		lbs	—	beats per minute	
WED		lbs	—	beats per minute	
THU		lbs	—	beats per minute	
FRI		lbs	—	beats per minute	
SAT		lbs	—	beats per minute	
SUN		lbs	—	beats per minute	

	Meds Taken (Y/N)	Daily Activity & Duration	Note if you are experiencing any symptoms listed on page 5: "When To Call Your Doctor"
MON			
TUE			
WED			
THU			
FRI			
SAT			
SUN			

WEEK OF:

	Date & Time	Today's Weight	B.P.	Heart Rate	Blood Sugar Measurements (mg/dL)
MON		lbs	—	beats per minute	
TUE		lbs	—	beats per minute	
WED		lbs	—	beats per minute	
THU		lbs	—	beats per minute	
FRI		lbs	—	beats per minute	
SAT		lbs	—	beats per minute	
SUN		lbs	—	beats per minute	

	Meds Taken (Y/N)	Daily Activity & Duration	Note if you are experiencing any symptoms listed on page 5: "When To Call Your Doctor"
MON			
TUE			
WED			
THU			
FRI			
SAT			
SUN			

WEEK OF:

	Date & Time	Today's Weight	B.P.	Heart Rate	Blood Sugar Measurements (mg/dL)
MON		lbs	—	beats per minute	
TUE		lbs	—	beats per minute	
WED		lbs	—	beats per minute	
THU		lbs	—	beats per minute	
FRI		lbs	—	beats per minute	
SAT		lbs	—	beats per minute	
SUN		lbs	—	beats per minute	

	Meds Taken (Y/N)	Daily Activity & Duration	Note if you are experiencing any symptoms listed on page 5: "When To Call Your Doctor"
MON			
TUE			
WED			
THU			
FRI			
SAT			
SUN			

WEEK OF:

	Date & Time	Today's Weight	B.P.	Heart Rate	Blood Sugar Measurements (mg/dL)
MON		lbs	—	beats per minute	
TUE		lbs	—	beats per minute	
WED		lbs	—	beats per minute	
THU		lbs	—	beats per minute	
FRI		lbs	—	beats per minute	
SAT		lbs	—	beats per minute	
SUN		lbs	—	beats per minute	

	Meds Taken (Y/N)	Daily Activity & Duration	Note if you are experiencing any symptoms listed on page 5: "When To Call Your Doctor"
MON			
TUE			
WED			
THU			
FRI			
SAT			
SUN			

WEEK OF:

	Date & Time	Today's Weight	B.P.	Heart Rate	Blood Sugar Measurements (mg/dL)
MON		lbs	—	beats per minute	
TUE		lbs	—	beats per minute	
WED		lbs	—	beats per minute	
THU		lbs	—	beats per minute	
FRI		lbs	—	beats per minute	
SAT		lbs	—	beats per minute	
SUN		lbs	—	beats per minute	

	Meds Taken (Y/N)	Daily Activity & Duration	Note if you are experiencing any symptoms listed on page 5: "When To Call Your Doctor"
MON			
TUE			
WED			
THU			
FRI			
SAT			
SUN			

WEEK OF:

	Date & Time	Today's Weight	B.P.	Heart Rate	Blood Sugar Measurements (mg/dL)
MON		lbs	—	beats per minute	
TUE		lbs	—	beats per minute	
WED		lbs	—	beats per minute	
THU		lbs	—	beats per minute	
FRI		lbs	—	beats per minute	
SAT		lbs	—	beats per minute	
SUN		lbs	—	beats per minute	

	Meds Taken (Y/N)	Daily Activity & Duration	Note if you are experiencing any symptoms listed on page 5: "When To Call Your Doctor"
MON			
TUE			
WED			
THU			
FRI			
SAT			
SUN			

WEEK OF:

	Date & Time	Today's Weight	B.P.	Heart Rate	Blood Sugar Measurements (mg/dL)
MON		lbs	—	beats per minute	
TUE		lbs	—	beats per minute	
WED		lbs	—	beats per minute	
THU		lbs	—	beats per minute	
FRI		lbs	—	beats per minute	
SAT		lbs	—	beats per minute	
SUN		lbs	—	beats per minute	

	Meds Taken (Y/N)	Daily Activity & Duration	Note if you are experiencing any symptoms listed on page 5: "When To Call Your Doctor"
MON			
TUE			
WED			
THU			
FRI			
SAT			
SUN			

WEEK OF:

	Date & Time	Today's Weight	B.P.	Heart Rate	Blood Sugar Measurements (mg/dL)
MON		lbs	—	beats per minute	
TUE		lbs	—	beats per minute	
WED		lbs	—	beats per minute	
THU		lbs	—	beats per minute	
FRI		lbs	—	beats per minute	
SAT		lbs	—	beats per minute	
SUN		lbs	—	beats per minute	

	Meds Taken (Y/N)	Daily Activity & Duration	Note if you are experiencing any symptoms listed on page 5: "When To Call Your Doctor"
MON			
TUE			
WED			
THU			
FRI			
SAT			
SUN			

Made in the USA
Las Vegas, NV
08 February 2021